I0435848

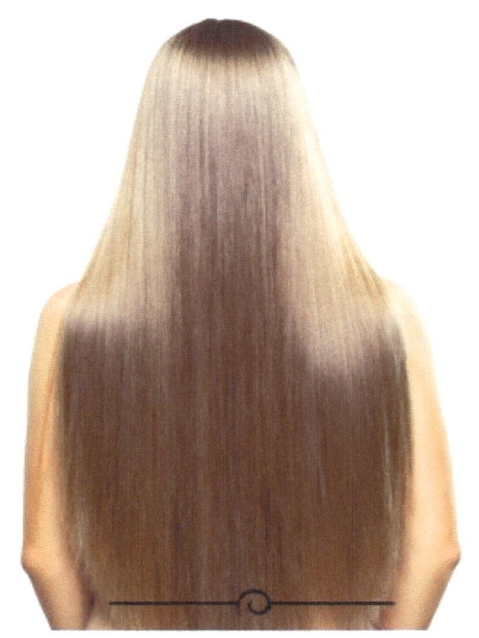

My New Healthy Hair

JOURNEY

By:

Jamie Wilkinson

TABLE OF CONTENTS

3

Introduction Of The Author

Wow! This is my first page and I can't even lie: I don't know where to start! I am a new mother with two beautiful children ages (3 and 5 years old) that I love dearly.

Apart from that, I have a degree in Mass Communication, completed several courses at Harvard University (Online), UMass-Amherst, etc.

I am also, a new social media personality that has been recognized and sponsored by many successful brands.

What can I say, "Life is good!"

Natural hair-- Oh Lord what a struggle!

I have been going natural officially from October 2015. I went natural before that then I gave into the temptation of relaxing my hair.

It doesn't hurt to try again -- and so I did!

In my new book, "My New Healthy Hair Journey" I am going to discuss my personal journey on life before and after my big chop and ten ways to keep your hair healthy and strong.

I don't want to bore you guys... so I am going to be brief and right to the point.

Once again thank you guys for supporting me and keep reading, keep viewing, keep supporting me!

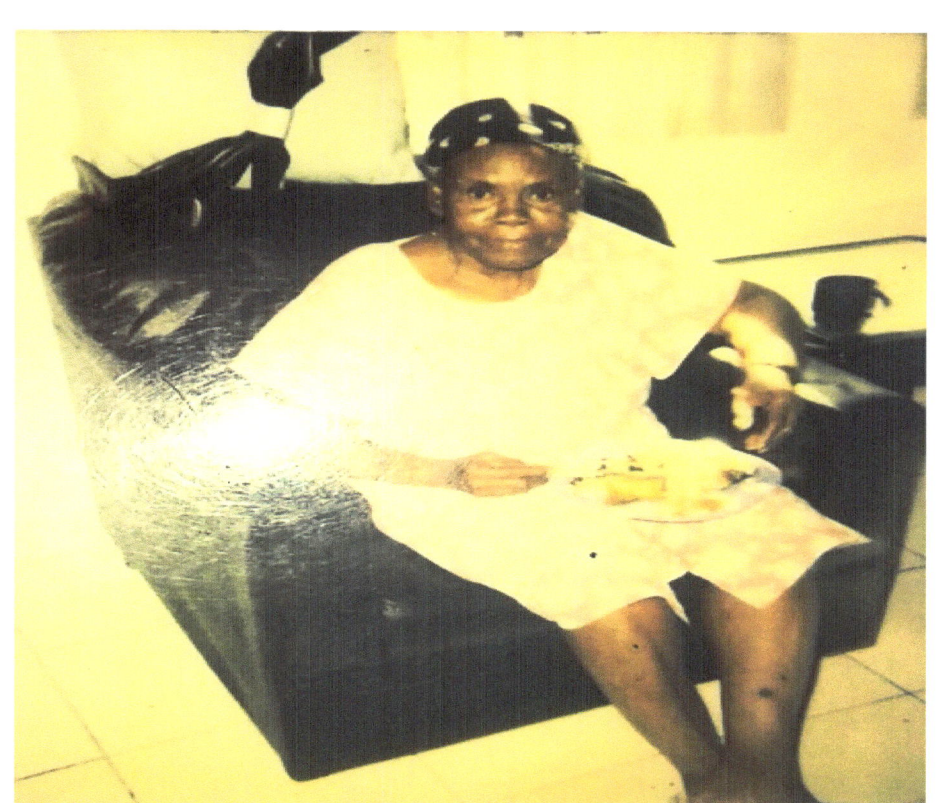

My Personal Journey

At first glance, I was grown up to hate wigs and anything not natural. I permed or relaxed my hair every month and then waited for new growth.

Don't get me wrong I am in no way bashing perms or relaxers at all okay. You have the right to change your mind at any point in this healthy hair journey.

Back to my story. So I always was frustrated with trying to keep my hair bone straight. It's like when I wash my hair the week after relaxing it-- it would revert right back to its original curl pattern.

My hair is and was very thick. Almost like it was resistant to relaxing and the only way to manipulate it was perming it!

Styling my hair was a struggle to say the least.

I could remember my grandmother breaking comb after comb after comb in my hair. It was absolutely ridiculous.

At that time, I just wanted my hair to look like everyone elses`!

WHEN I STOPPED PERMING MY HAIR

In the year 2015 I soon decided to stop with the perming. I didn't want to stop wearing my hair straight-- there's a difference!

One week turned into a month then a month turned into six months. I was so proud of myself. But let's face it-- styling it was just too much at times.

I grew tired of smelling burnt hair and so I relaxed it. And then, just like every other time it began reverting back to the same frizzy mess.

Not to mention, I had several textures going on-- that just looked weird!

Then in the beginning of October 2015, I did a silicone treatment and that was it. My ends became so darn stringy-- I had to big chop!

Right before that my little sister let me do a big chop on her hair. Then I became inspired to do the same.

Thank God for wigs. They literally saved my life!

THE SHAME

Oh my gosh! There was such a range of emotion going on when I cut my hair that short.

On one hand, I felt happy, accomplished and then on the other I felt ashamed, and perhaps criticized.

Don't misinterpret what I am saying. I am proud of my curl pattern. However, the large quantity of my hair was gone!

My- crown- of- glory was reduced!

Sigh!

I couldn't even wear my hair in a ponytail!

I just wanted to hide and not let anyone see me that way at all!

The Strength

After a few weeks I built up enough strength to be happy about it again. And after a few months it even started growing faster than before.

This time I implemented biotin, collagen and vitamin C supplements into my diet and I drank more water.

Also, I changed my styling practices.

For example, I used heat protectant and blow dried my hair straight before flat ironing it.

That way I minimized the amount of times I passed the flat iron through my hair.

I reflected on all the silly things that I did to my hair and I improved on them!

Eventually my hair started growing back enough to style. Yay! I like(d) that!

EXTERNAL REACTIONS

I can't really say anything really bad about what everyone thought about my hair because I always wear wigs.

What I can say was that there were several harmless jokes made. LOL!

I watched parodies of men`s reactions to their significant others transition.

I know that my head had a weird shape and that's why I always tried to balance that out with my hair or weave.

I even joined natural hair communities and laughed at myself a few times.

Tempted To Texturize My Hair

So there are persons out there that somehow believe that texturizing one's hair is still having natural hair?

So I did my research and discovered that texturizing is a form of mild relaxer. At this point in the game, I thought to myself. Hmmm I have come this far, why would I chemically treat my hair with perm again?

Don't get me wrong. You can relax, texturize or perm your hair if you want. You have the freedom to do so.

I on the other hand just want my hair free from chemicals because it grows so much faster.

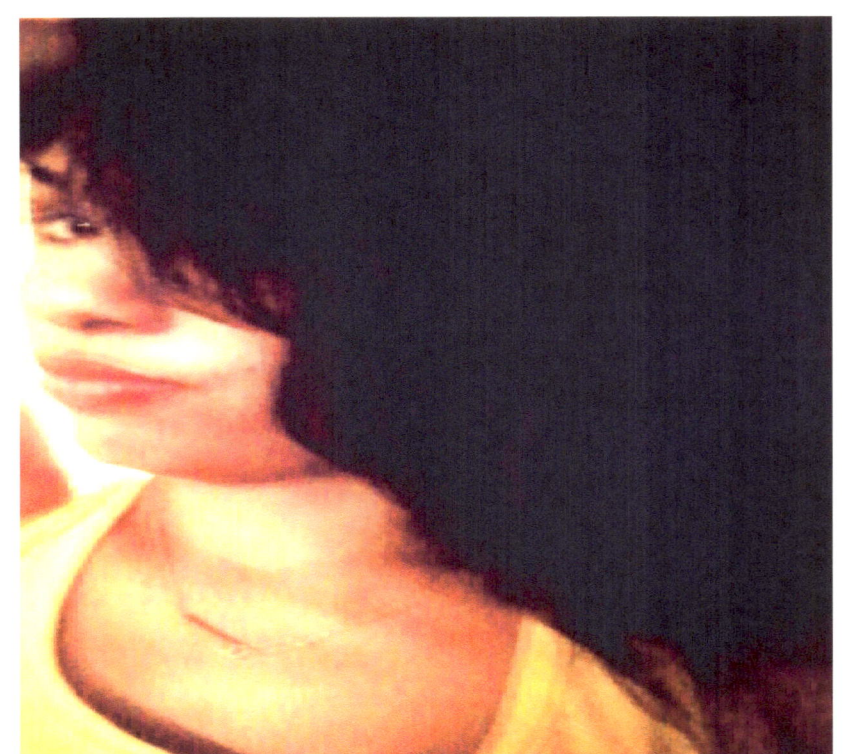

AM I SEXY?

Am I sexy with natural hair?

Umm? Heck yeah! But seriously, there were times when my femininity was questioned.

I just didn't feel like my regular self.

Imagine wearing your hair a certain way then boom change?

I couldn't quite understand it, then I started to adjust. Especially after my hair became neck length.

In essence, I just wanted my hair back in a way. Now I have discovered the awesome option of wearing wigs and weaves.

WEARING WEAVE IS AWESOME

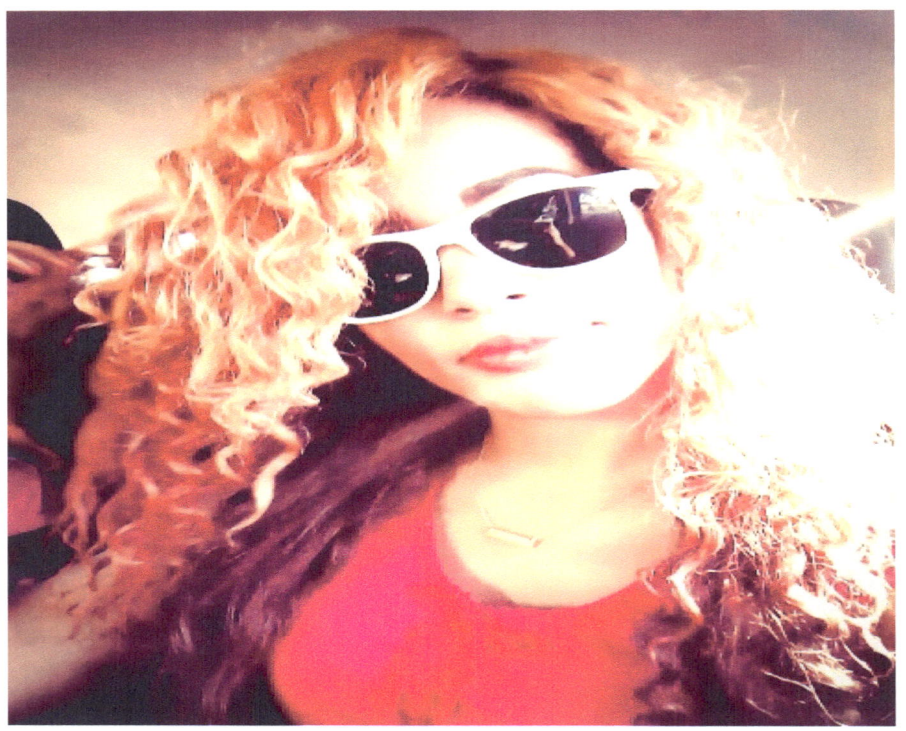

Can I tell you: weaves saved my life!

First of all:

1. I have a big head

2. My head has an odd shape

3. Short cuts don't suit me

4. I look better with long, voluminous hair

With that being said. Weave is awesome and it solved all my problems. Every female wants to feel confident and complete and hair can do that for you!

HUMIDITY

My hair has always been prone to humidity. Only one way I could avoid the elements and that was to wear wigs.

I could just finish styling my hair and my hair could be very smooth and frizz free then as soon as the moisture in the air hits my hair -- ping, my hair forms a frizzy ball of hair, no curls or nothing-- just frizz.

At times, I don't even care. I just throw on a wig that's it!

Hair Moisture

One of the best ways to retain moisture is protective styling. A lot of people do it and you wouldn't even know!

Other ways to trap moisture in your hair is to learn it's porosity. Then work from there!

You should always try to learn the chemistry of your hair. What works for me doesn't mean that it would work for you.

For me, my hair thrives on Aunt Jackie's. I condition, oil, seal and braid my hair and then install or put on a wig/unit.

Bad Hair Days

Bad hair days! Blah! Who needs them!. To be real, everyday while being natural has the potential to be one.

In actuality, you can't let it get you down.

You've got to find a new found confidence to be able to rock that hairstyle with a smile. But make sure it looks good though!

Natural hair can look beautiful!

MYTHS

People that cut their hair enjoy what it looks like

People that go natural are Afrocentric

People that cut their hair have a easy time styling it

People that cut their hair always grow long hair

Realistically,we may never know why a person may cut their hair. Factually, it is easy to say that one`s hair journey depends on genetics.

Whether or not your genetic predisposition is equipped with everything that you want your hair to be.

Personally, I have accepted that my hair is not going to be the longest, finest, or the curliest.

I can definitely find other ways to enhance my hair's appearance! My hair is good just the way it is!

Real Reasons I Went Natural

Reasons why I went natural:

- longer hair

- healthier hair

- healthier scalp

- less chemicals

- hair length challenge

- wanted to try something new for a change; staying consistent

Ten Steps To Keep Your Healthy

1. Wash your hair often

2. Condition your hair after shampooing

3. Deep condition your hair

4. Use minimal heat to prevent breakage

5. Use a Denman brush or wide tooth comb and detangle from your ends up to your roots

6. Oil and seal your ends

7. Use protective styles as often as possible

8. Be gentle while styling your natural hair

9. Drink lots of water

10. Take your hair vitamins

WASH YOUR HAIR OFTEN

Always wash your hair often. You need a clean scalp for your hair to grow. Use a shampoo that is free of sulfates and parabens like Aunt Jackie's.

Caution: don't wash it too much though, you don't want your hair to become brittle and break off.

CONDITION YOUR HAIR AFTER SHAMPOOING

After washing your hair it may become drier than usual. Use a conditioner that is moisturizing and suitable for your hair texture.

Conditioned hair retains length and moisture.

DEEP CONDITION YOUR HAIR

There are instances where your hair is going to need a deep conditioner. I use a hair bonnet as well so that I can lock in all the essential moisture that my hair needs.

Use Minimal Heat

Use less heat to avoid hair breakage. Try to use a heat protectant as much as possible. And if you blow dry your hair on warm or hot always use cool air when you are done to close the hair shaft.

OIL AND SEAL YOUR ENDS

Oil and seal your ends to avoid splitting. You can also oil your scalp. Jojoba and Almond oil are great!

If you want you can also dust your ends.

10 Steps continued

Use protective styles as often as possible- this would include braiding, twisting, etc.

Be gentle while styling your hair/ minimize styling- try not to make too much contact with your hair

Drink plenty of water- water keeps the blood and nutrients flowing throughout the body; your hair needs this

Take your hair vitamins- biotin, collagen and vitamin c all help your hair to grow

AUNT JACKIE'S

My hair responded very well to this brand and I advise curly girls like myself to use Aunt Jackie's in their hair.

It was like my hair was so hungry and thirsty for their products. I think if my hair could smile it was smiling each time I used them.

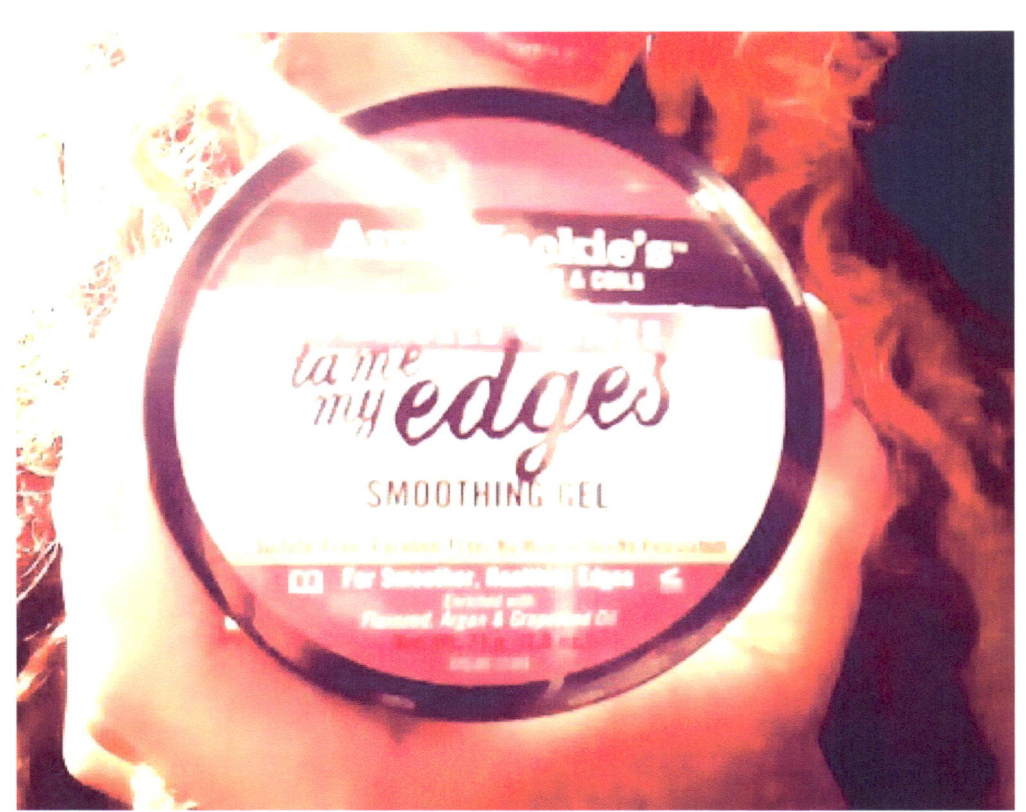

GARNIER FRUCTIS

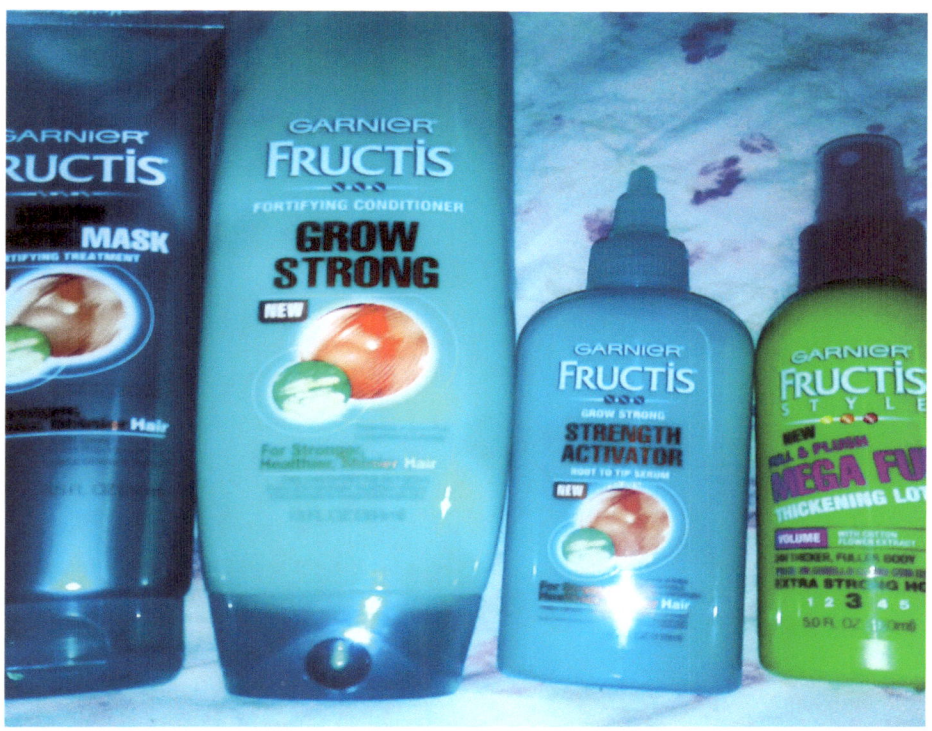

Garnier Fructis is really a good brand if you want longer, stronger hair. I have tried this brand off and on for the last 15 years and it really does work!

HAIR SENTIMENTS

All I can say is I love my hair and now that I really think about it I wouldn't change it for the world!

CONCLUSION

Honestly, natural , healthy hair is truly a journey. Only the strong can survive and persevere through it all. Attaining this goal takes time and dedication.

And believe me when you get it-- you are going to be so happy!

Just set realistic hair goals and accomplish them one step at a time.

Change your thinking and be nice to your hair!

MY BEAUTIFUL DAUGHTER

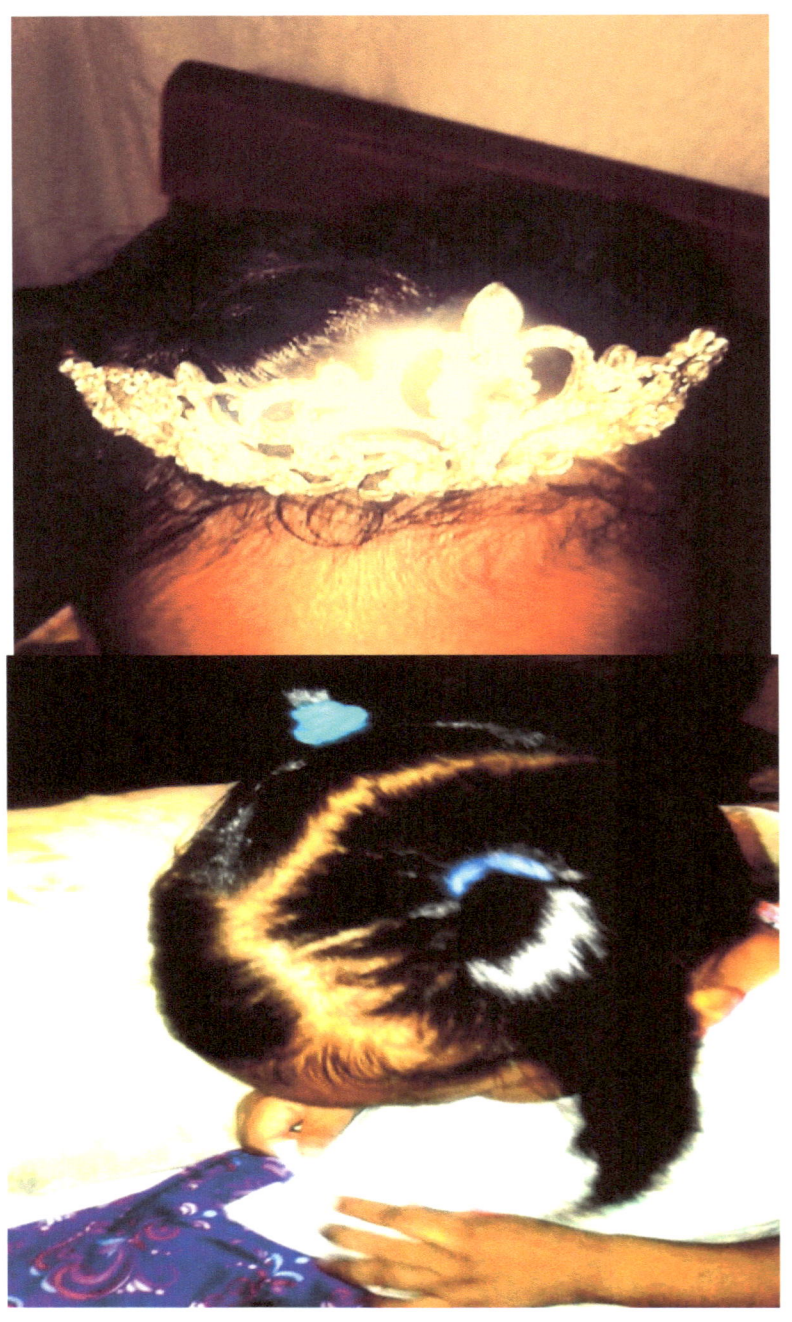

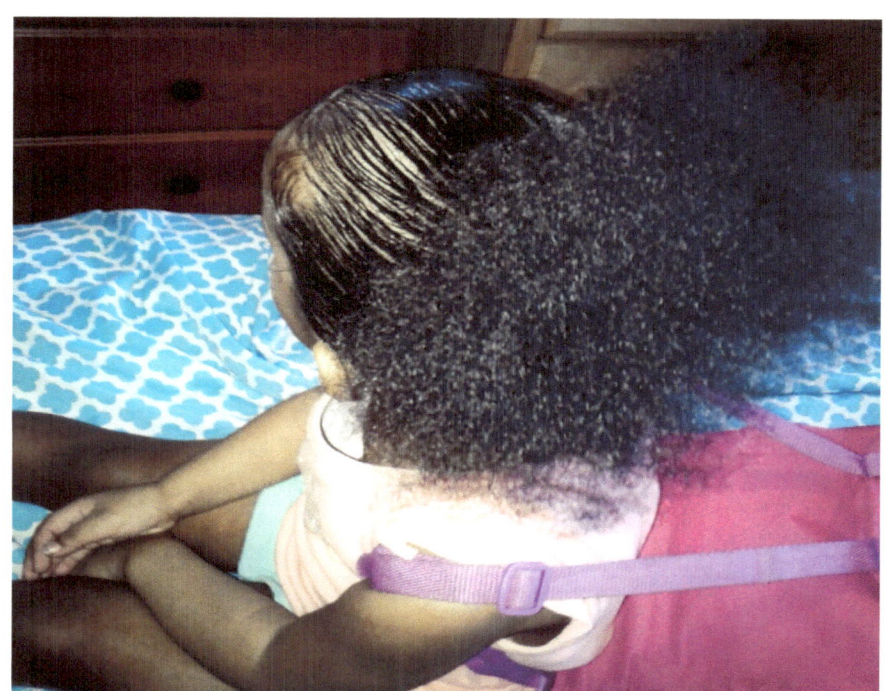

www.ingramcontent.com/pod-product-compliance
Lightning Source LLC
Chambersburg PA
CBHW060840290526
45792CB00006BB/2004